ANCIENT FOOD, MODERN MEDICINE

Olive oil has been a cornerstone of the Mediterranean diet since the Bronze Age. Today the ancient tradition has been validated by modern medical research, which has established it as a truly "friendly fat." Olive oil is heart-healthy, containing monounsaturated fatty acids and other nutrients that protect against cardiovascular disease. Olive oil reduces the risk of breast and colon cancer, promotes gallbladder function and is being used to treat arthritis. Best of all, it improves the taste and enjoyment of foods while replacing fats that are detrimental to your health.

ABOUT THE AUTHOR

Jean Barilla is a medical writer, editor and health media consultant with B.A. and M.S. degrees in biology from New York University and a B.S. in Basic Medical Sciences from the University of South Alabama College of Medicine, has taught medical students and been a staff biologist for the Food and Drug Administration. She has written many articles for scientific and popular publications, edits a nutritional newsletter for physicians, and compiled the *Nutrition Superbooks* (*The Antioxidants* and *The Good Fats and Oils*) for Keats Publishing, where she is an editor. She is host of "Entertaining Health," a weekly radio program on AM 850 WREF in Fairfield County, Connecticut.

Olive Oil Miracle

How the Mediterranean marvel helps protect against arthritis, heart disease and breast cancer

Jean Barilla, M.S.

Keats Publishing, Inc. New Canaan, Connecticut

Acknowledgment
Many thanks to the International Olive Oil Council for providing informative literature on the history of olive oil and on regulatory matters affecting standards of olive oil production.

Olive Oil Miracle is intended solely for informational and educational purposes, and not as medical advice. Please consult a medical or health professional if you have questions about your health.

OLIVE OIL MIRACLE

Copyright © 1996 by Jean Barilla, M.S.

All Rights Reserved

No part of this book may be reproduced in any form without the written consent of the publisher.

ISBN: 0-87983-763-2

Printed in the United States of America

02 03 04 05 RCP 10 9 8 7 6 5 4 3

CONTENTS

Introduction 6
The Immortal Tree 7
A Fat by Any Other Name 11
Fat Metabolism 14
Olive Oil and Disease: Research
     Confirms Tradition..21
Olive Oil in the Diet..28
How Good Is the Oil?..34
Green Gold Goodness to Purified Perfection..............41
Olive Oil Facts 43
Summary 45
Resources...45
References 46

INTRODUCTION

If you want to choose a fat source in your diet that will protect you against heart disease and breast cancer, help your digestive system function properly and be useful in treating arthritis and diabetes, olive oil will meet those needs and more.

Olive oil, this good fat, will also enhance the taste of your food and leave you more satiated, especially when dieting. Whether olive oil is used in cooking or as a condiment or even in baking, adding this health-friendly fat will please your palate.

There is increasing evidence that low-fat diets are detrimental to your health because these diets omit or significantly reduce the intake of essential fatty acids and other good fats that are necessary for normal body metabolism and optimal health. The good fats and oils are even needed in order for your body to *burn* fats.

Olive oil contains fats that can make up for the deficiencies of essential fatty acids caused by poor eating habits or low-fat diets. The fats in olive oil can be used by the body to make energy and to keep arteries flexible. Olive oil fats also protect genetic material from attacks by toxic chemicals.

A diet that omits or reduces levels of the "bad" fats, and includes olive oil, the superstar of the good fats, will be palatable, satisfying and a giant step in the direction of optimal health and personal enjoyment.

THE IMMORTAL TREE

The olive oil tree and its fruit have been entwined in the epic of human social and scientific development for over 6,000 years. According to Greek mythology, the goddess Athena gave two great gifts to her people: wisdom and—because wisdom cannot be eaten—the olive. A cornerstone of the Mediterranean economy, olive oil has been used as a fuel, in soap and cosmetics, during religious ceremonies and most importantly, as a therapeutic agent. Before 400 B.C., Hippocrates, the "father of medicine," prescribed olive oil for curing ulcers, cholera, gallbladder problems and muscular pains. Today, science and medicine can verify that the health benefits claimed by our ancestors were indeed true.

The olive tree is a member of the family Oleacaea, which also includes the privet, lilac, ash, forsythia and jasmine. The origin of the edible olive, *Olea europaea*, precedes recorded history, but undoubtedly it is one of the world's oldest cultivated crops. It was an olive leaf that Noah's dove took back to the Ark.

OLIVE OIL TIME LINE

- Pliocene era (1,000,000+ years ago)—olive leaves fossilized in what is now Mongardino, Italy.
- Upper Paleolithic (750,000-15,000 years ago)—fossilized remains of olives found in North Africa.
- 6,000 years ago—cultivation of olives in the Mediterranean basin.
- Bronze Age (up to 8th century B.C.)—pieces of wild olive trees and stones from this era found in Spain.
- 16th century B.C.—Phoenicians disseminated the olive throughout the Greek isles.
- 14th and 12th centuries B.C.—cultivation of olives on the Greek mainland.

- 6th century B.C.—spread of cultivation throughout Mediterranean countries, to Sicily and to southern Italy.
- 600 B.C.—olive cultivation introduced in Marseilles, France.
- 600 B.C. to 1492 A.D.—after expanding throughout the Mediterranean, olive farming spread to the Americas.

OLIVE OIL IN HISTORY, LEGEND AND RELIGION

The first olive trees were carried from Seville, Spain to the West Indies and later to the North and South America. By 1560, olive groves were being cultivated in Mexico, Peru, California, Chile and Argentina, where one of the plants brought over during the Conquest—the old Arauco olive tree—lives to this day. Now the olive tree is farmed in Africa, Australia, Japan and China.

Because the olive tree offers life, food, and protection, it has been immortalized in legends, religion and ancient literature. Shedding and replacing its leaves every year, it symbolizes longevity, fertility and maturity. According to legend, Adam, when close to death, invoked the word of the Lord who had given him the oil of mercy for his redemption and that of all mankind. Adam sent his son Seth to beseech the cherub that watched over the mountain where the Garden of Eden stood. The cherub took three seeds from the tree of knowledge of good and evil and told Seth to place them in the mouth of Adam, once he was dead. When Adam was buried on Mount Tabor the three seeds germinated, sending out roots. Later, three stems formed an olive tree, a cedar and a cypress—the three trees of the Mediterranean.

Six thousand years ago, the Egyptians credited Isis, the wife of Osiris, the supreme god of Egypt, with teaching the cultivation and uses of the olive.

The Greeks had many legends involving the olive tree. The naming of the city of Athens, Greece was the most famous story. As mentioned above, the goddess of peace and wisdom and daughter of Zeus, Pallas Athena, was the source of the olive tree. When a small colony was founded in Attica in the 17th century B.C., the inhabitants of the area, who had been nomads, wanted a name for their town. Athena and Poseidon (the god of the waters, earthquakes and horses) disputed the honor of naming the town. The gods agreed to set up a contest and grant that honor to whichever of the two contestants provided the most useful invention.

Poseidon struck the ground with his trident and brought forth a magnificent horse, "beautiful, swift, capable of pulling heavy chariots and winning in combat." Athena made sprout an olive tree "capable of giving a flame for lighting up the night, of soothing wounds, of being a precious food both rich in flavor and a source of energy." The people chose the olive tree as the invention of greater use. Athena was granted sovereignty over the region and over the city which bears her name.

The olive tree that sprouted in the Acropolis in Athens was surrounded by a wall and was guarded by warriors who were consecrated to its defense. When enemies approached, all the citizens gathered inside the city walls, near the olive tree, until danger had passed. Later, during the Median wars and after the burning of the Acropolis and its sacred olive tree by Xerxes, the Athenians returned to their city. The monuments were destroyed, but the olive tree planted by the goddess had sent out new roots, overcoming destruction and earning itself the symbol of immortality.

The Greeks attributed the cultivation and use of the olive tree to Aristaeus, the son of Apollo and the nymph Cyrene. Only virgins and chaste men were entrusted with tending olive groves.

> **Insider commodity trading, Greek style:**
> In Greece about 600 B.C., Thales of Miletus predicted from observing the stars that oil production was going to be extraordinary in the next season. He leased the region's mills and through his monopoly earned a fabulous profit. He was one of the first people to trade in oil.

The Romans had their own legends about olive oil (and a popular saying: "The necessary ingredients of civilization are wine and olive oil"). They believed that Romulus and Remus, the descendants of the gods (who were raised by a wolf) and founders of Rome, saw the light of day for the first time beneath the branches of an olive tree. In Roman mythology, Minerva, goddess of peace and wisdom (the Roman version of Athena), is said to have given the gifts of olive cultivation and wool-spinning to mankind. Hercules was said to be the instigator of the olive's expansion along the shores of the Mediterranean. The legend relates that every time he struck the ground with his olive club, it sent out roots and an olive tree sprang up.

The Bible is a rich source of information on the religious and culinary uses of olive oil. In Genesis, as mentioned above, the dove set free by Noah returned to the Ark in the evening with a small green olive branch in its beak. This was a sign of the abating of the Flood and a symbol of reestablished peace between God and man.

The Book of Judges states, "The trees once went forth to anoint a king over them, and they said to the olive tree, 'Reign over us'. But the olive tree said to them, "Shall I leave my fatness by which God and men are honored, and go to wave over the trees?" In Exodus, the Lord tells Moses, "Send your children to bring you the most virgin of oils from the olive tree, so that it is always burning in the lamp." In the first Book of Kings, Hiram, King of Tyre, supplies Solomon with as much cedar and fir wood as was needed to build the Temple and Solomon gives him wheat and virgin olive oil in return.

The olive tree was an exceptional witness to the life of Jesus. In the Garden of Gethsemane on the Mount of Olives, Jesus prayed and wept immediately before his crucifixion and death, and was buried amongst olive groves.

In the Koran, there is reference to the tree "that sprouts on Mount Sinai and provides oil as a condiment to the table." The Koran exalts Allah and his light in these words: "Allah is the light of the heavens and the earth. His light may be compared to a niche that enshrines a lamp, the lamp within a crystal of star-like brilliance. It is lit from a blessed olive tree neither eastern nor western."

Greek and Roman literature makes many references to the olive. Homer comments on the gentle radiance of oil in lamps. The Greeks say that Leto gave birth in the shade of an olive tree during her stay at Delos. An olive branch was also a symbol of supplicants and of those seeking a truce and peace.

Virgil praises the olive tree and its oily fruit in the *Georgics*.. In his *Metamorphoses*, Ovid portrays Baucis as preparing a frugal meal with olive oil for his celestial guests. Horace, Lucretius, Martial and most other Roman poets mentioned "the silvery tree."

In his treatise *On Agriculture* Cato lists the material necessary for growing olive trees and producing the oil. Pliny the Elder observes in his *Natural History* that rainfall at the time the olive tree is in bloom is the most unfortunate accident, since this causes the fruit to drop. Pliny also refers to the oil that keeps teeth white and cures diseased gums.

Columella in his *Treatise on Agriculture* states that "of all the trees, it is the one that incurs the least expense, even though it is the first in importance." In his 2000-year-old cookbook *On Cooking* Apicius constantly mentions olive oil from Spain.

All the civilizations that have cultivated and used olive oil sing its praises. In many cases, their health and their lives have depended on this gift from the gods.

Despite the extensive history and usage of olive oil in other countries, in North America, today, olives are mostly known as a garnish. Only in the last decade has extra virgin olive oil become readily available. Knowledge of the health-giving and healing properties of olive oil are just now opening the eyes of the modern medical community. Where ancient wisdom and cutting-edge science meet, we have found a pot of gold . . . green gold.

The olive tree lasts and bears its fruit for centuries. It can grow to 40 feet tall and the wood is resistant to decay. The tree can tolerate drought periods of five or six months through the summer, provided winter rainfall is at least 8 to 10 inches. The trees are usually unirrigated, but will use just as much water as other trees if it is available. The olive can endure adverse conditions which would kill most other fruit trees. The tree, even when cut down, will bring forth new growth from its roots for future generations—truly a miracle.

The olive tree, an evergreen, can live to 600 years or more, with some specimens reportedly being over 1,000 years old. The tree must be 5-8 years old before it will bear fruit, but full production is not reached until 15 or 20 years.

A FAT BY ANY OTHER NAME. . .

In order to better understand the health benefits of olive oil it is helpful to know "fat terminology." Fats, oils, lipids, fatty acids, saturated and mono- and polyunsaturated fats, trans fatty acids, to name a few—what do these terms mean?

THE BASICS—KEY FATS AND RELATED MOLECULES

Just what is fat? Fat is one of the nutrients required for life and health, along with proteins, carbohydrates, vitamins, minerals and water. Another name for "fat" is "lipid." What we call "fat" is a lipid that is solid at room temperature; oil is a lipid that is liquid at room temperature.

The building blocks of fats and oils are called fatty acids. "Fatty" indicates that one end of the fat or oil molecule does not dissolve in water, while "acid" refers to the other end of the molecule that does dissolve in water.

Fatty acids are made up of atoms of carbon (C), hydrogen (H) and oxygen (O) linked together like chains.

When the chain of carbon atoms has as many hydrogen atoms as it can possibly hold, and only has single bonds between the carbon atoms, the fat is called saturated. These fats are solid at room temperature. The greater the saturated fat content, the higher will be the temperature required to melt the fat. Animal fats and two vegetable fats (oil from coconuts and palm kernels) are highly saturated. For most people, a diet high in saturated fat stimulates the liver to make "bad" low-density lipoprotein (LDL) cholesterol (more about this later). The saturated molecules have a tendency to stick together. An excess can cause heart and blood vessel health problems.

When the chain has fewer hydrogen atoms, and double bonds between the carbon atoms, the fat is unsaturated. Unsaturated fats will stay liquid in cold temperatures. Unsaturated fats tend to be anti-sticky and move apart, and are more fluid. A monounsaturated fat is an unsaturated fat that has one carbon=carbon (C=C) double bond. Some examples of monounsaturated fats are olive, canola, peanut and avocado oils. Polyunsaturated fats have two or more double bonds between carbons; examples are corn, soy, sesame, sunflower and safflower oils.

> Epidemiological studies have shown that diets in which monounsaturated fatty acids are the predominant fat source are also the best diets for heart health. Olive oil is a highly monounsaturated fat.

To complicate things further, double bonds come in two types: cis and trans configurations. To understand what this terminology means, you first need to know that the actual fat molecules are three-dimensional and that bonds project in all directions from carbon atoms. An analogy would be a child's Tinker Toy set with the rods (bonds) sticking out in all directions from the rounded connecting pieces (atoms). When both hydrogen atoms on the carbons involved in the double bond are on the same side of the molecule, the conformation is called "cis" (Latin for "on this side"). When the hydrogens are on opposite sides of the C=C bond, the conformation is called "trans" ("on the other side").

The trans form makes the fat more stable (less likely to become rancid) than the cis form. This artificial transformation is fine for extending the shelf life of products containing fats, but it is harmful to your health. Even though trans fats are unsaturated, they behave like saturated fats and are associated with all the harmful effects of the saturated fats.

The numbering system for fat molecules assigns numbers to carbon atoms starting from the methyl end. This method of numbering is called the omega system. Plant sources of fatty acids contain omega-3 and omega-6 forms, where the number indicates where the double bond is located.

The essential fatty acids (EFAs), those that we cannot make and must obtain from foods, are linoleic acid (an omega-6 form) and alpha-linolenic acid (an omega-3 form).

FROM GOOD TO BAD

Hydrogenation is the most common way of changing healthful natural oils into products that can have major detrimental effects on our health. It is done by industry for one reason, to save money. Hydrogenated oils have a longer shelf life. Manufacturers can start with cheap, low quality oils and turn them into margarines that may fool your palate but not your body.

Hydrogenation is actually the process of creating unnatural sources of saturated fat. This is done by adding hydrogen atoms to the carbon atoms in the fat. This chemical process uses aluminum, a metal associated with Alzheimer's disease (a degenerative disease of the brain resulting in mental disability and eventually death).

The fat can be completely hydrogenated—all of the double bonds in an oil are saturated with hydrogen. In this case, there are no cis or trans forms since there are no double bonds left. This process produces unnatural fatty acid fragments and other altered molecules, some of which may be toxic. The long-term effects of these substances are unknown. Hydrogenated fats include margarine, solid vegetable shortening and all processed foods made with partially hydrogenated oils.

Partial hydrogenation, where there are still some double bonds, results in fats that have both cis and trans molecules. Trans fatty acids interfere with body biochemistry. While the body can make cell membranes and hormones from cis fatty acids, it is not known what is done with the trans forms. Trans fatty acids have been shown to increase LDL (the "bad") cholesterol levels, and decrease the "good" high-density lipoprotein (HDL) cholesterol. Trans fatty acids also interfere with the detoxification system in the liver and affect essential fatty acid metabolism.

According to an article in the *Harvard Heart Letter*,[1] new data indicate that the effects of trans fatty acids on cholesterol levels increase a person's risk of heart attack. Even small amounts of trans fatty acids can be harmful. In the Nurse's Health Study, it was found that women who ate four or more teaspoons of margarine per day had a 66 percent increase in the risk of heart attack when compared to those who ate margarine less than once a month. In the average margarine, the amount of trans fatty acids is between 1 percent and 30 percent of the total fat content.

Based on the data, the Harvard newsletter said that experts suggest that consumers be wary of partially hydrogenated oils and minimize use of both butter and margarine. "Cook with olive or canola oil and avoid deep-fried food" was the message.

FAT METABOLISM

Saturated fatty acids are mainly used as fuel that our body "burns" to produce energy. Burning in this sense means that the chemical energy stored in the fatty acids is released as a result of complex chemical reactions that go on in the body. When we take in too many calories, our body stores the excess as fat to prevent the metabolic "fire" from getting too hot.

Monounsaturated fatty acids can also be used to produce energy. When the body is low in essential fatty acids, the monounsaturated fats can be converted and partially perform the function of these essential fats. We burn essential fatty acids for energy only when there is an excess. They are better used to make phospholipids for the cell membranes and take part in many vital biological processes. For additional information on fat metabolism see:my *Nutrition Superbook. Volume 2. The Good Fats and Oils*, (Keats Publishing, Inc., 1996).

Olive oil, although it contains only small amounts of the essential fatty acids, linoleic and alpha-linolenic acid, has beneficial effects on health. These health benefits result from the other components in the oil. Olive oil contains about 75 percent of the non-essential monounsaturated fatty acid, oleic acid. Oleic acid is a member of the omega-9 family.

Oleic acid is also found in almond, peanut, pistachio, pecan, canola, avocado, hazelnut, cashew, and macadamia oils, as well as in plant and animal cells. This fatty acid helps keep our arteries flexible, reducing the risk of heart disease. Oleic acid as well as linoleic acid and alpha-linolenic acid are also antimutagenic. This means that they can protect our genetic material from being attacked and altered by toxic chemicals.

In addition to the benefits of monounsaturation discussed above, there are also minor components in olive oil that enhance its health-giving properties. Olive oil contains substances that have healing and anti-inflammatory effects; among these are phenolic compounds with antioxidant properties. Olive oil also contains several minor but important components: the antioxidants beta-carotene and tocopherols (vitamin E family), and chlorophyll. Chlorophyll is rich in magnesium. Patients with cardiovascular disease are often magnesium deficient. Chlorophyll is also found in other unrefined green oils such as hemp, pumpkin and avocado.

Two tablespoons of olive oil supply approximately 3.2 mg of vitamin E—approximately the amount in a quarter cup of mixed nuts. Other vegetable oils may have more vitamin E. These oils, however, are also high in polyunsaturated fatty acids (PUFA), which are associated with a higher risk of developing certain cancers.

Vitamin E is expressed in milligrams (mg) of d-alpha-tocopherol: 1 mg d-alpha-tocopherol = 1.5 International Units (IU)
1 mg dl-alpha-tocopherol = 1.0 IU

Some researchers believe that the ratio of vitamin E to PUFA in an oil is a better measure of its health value than simply measuring vitamin E alone. Olive oil has a very low PUFA content, and thus has a vitamin E/PUFA ratio higher than soybean, corn, sunflower, and cottonseed oils.

Other compounds found in olive oil include tyrosol and hydroxytyrosol, phenolic compounds derived from the olive pulp.[2] When these phenolics are added to other oils, they have an antioxidant effect.

Squalene, a precursor of phytosterols, is another component of olive oil. Phytosterols protect against cholesterol absorption from foods. This substance helps deliver oxygen to tissues, especially those short of oxygen. It also increases heart activity, dilates blood vessels and inhibits atherosclerosis. Squalene is also very active and effective in the rehabilitation of scars. Olive oil also contains phytosterols such as beta-sitosterol, which as mentioned, can protect against cholesterol absorption, thus lowering cholesterol levels.

Polyphenols, plant compounds with antioxidant abilities, help stabilize the oil and are in part responsible for its color. Research is now under way to determine the health effects of these compounds.

Triterpenic substances, which are modified sterols, are also found in olive oil. These include several groups of compounds: triterphenethyl alcohols, monohydroxy and dihydroxy triterpenes, and triterpenic alcohols. Included in these groups are cycloartenol, alpha-and beta-amyrin, 24-methylene-cycloartenol, and erythrodiol. Hydroxy triterpenic acids such as oleanolic, maslinic and ursolic acids are also found in olive oil. The chemical structures of these substances indicate that they are good candidates for being credited with the cardiovascular benefits of olive oil. Triterpenic acids also have anti-inflammatory effects. Very little research has as yet been done on these substances.[3]

THE MUFAS AND THE PUFAS

The controversy over the effects of monounsaturated (MUFA) and polyunsaturated (PUFA) fatty acids on cholesterol is still an open issue. Olive oil is rich in MUFA and you will learn in this section how these fatty acids redeem "bad" cholesterol and keep you safe.

In the 1960s, researchers noted that MUFA and carbohydrates did not affect plasma cholesterol levels. The PUFA were found to lower total plasma cholesterol and low density lipoprotein (LDL) cholesterol (the "bad" cholesterol). So, it was recommended that PUFA replace saturated fatty acids in the diet. However, that wasn't the whole story. PUFA was also found to lower high-density lipoprotein (HDL) cholesterol (the "good" cholesterol) and high intake was implicated in increasing susceptibility to gallstones and cancer that was induced by chemical substances.

Later studies found that both MUFA or PUFA decreased LDL cholesterol. Because of the lack of evidence of the safety of high PUFA diets, and the negative effect on HDL, MUFA was instead recommended to replace dietary saturated fatty acids. Although there was subsequent data to indicate that a diet balanced in amounts of MUFA and PUFA would have similar beneficial effects, other effects of MUFA tipped the scales in favor of increasing dietary MUFA. Among these findings was the fact that plasma cholesterol levels are lower in countries with a high content of oleic acid (the major fatty acid in olive oil), present in the diet.

> Cholesterol is a fat or lipid and is not soluble in water. For it to be transported through blood, a watery liquid, it must be bound to proteins. These complexes of cholesterol and protein are called "lipoproteins."

MUFA were found to be better dietary components for non-insulin-dependent diabetics than low-fat, high carbohydrate diets. The reason is that there is also a triglyceride-lowering affect associated with MUFA in the diet. Blood pressure-lowering effects were also found when diets were high in oleic acid.

Olive oil contains mainly nonessential monounsaturated fatty acids with small amounts of the essential fatty acids, linoleic and alpha-linolenic acids. Both essential and nonessential fatty acids in olive oil contribute to its therapeutic effects.

Olive oil contains the following MUFA:

- Linoleic acid (omega-6) 3.5 percent to 20 percent (average 10 percent)
- alpha-linolenic (omega-3) 0.1 percent to .6 percent
- oleic acid (omega-9) 63 percent to 83 percent (average 75 percent)

- palmitoleic acid (omega-7) 0.5 percent to 3 percent (average 2 percent)

Oleic acid increases the incorporation of omega-3 fatty acids into cell membranes, thus maintaining the fluidity and function of this cell structure. When the membranes around cells remain fluid or soft, essential nutrients can get into cells more easily. Products that the cells make, such as proteins and hormones, can get out more easily as well.

One of the problems associated with aging is a stiffening of the cell membrane. Cells in this state cannot function at optimal levels. If cells are not functioning properly, then the organs that these cells are made of also cannot function properly. If the organs do not function properly, the logical result is that a person does not live as long, and the quality of life is diminished. A seemingly small problem, lack of membrane fluidity, therefore has far reaching consequences.

Oleic acid also decreases the oxidation of LDL cholesterol. This action reduces the atherogenic potential of the LDL (see below).

Linoleic acid, a component of olive oil and an omega-6 essential fatty acid, is one of the two main fats we must obtain from foods in order to be healthy. Signs of deficiency of linoleic acid include:

- eczema-like skin eruptions
- loss of hair
- liver degeneration
- behavioral disturbances
- kidney degeneration
- excessive water loss through the skin and thirst
- drying up of glands
- susceptibility to infection
- failure of wound healing
- sterility in men
- miscarriage in females
- arthritis-like conditions
- heart and circulatory problems
- growth retardation

A prolonged absence of linoleic acid from the diet is fatal. All of the deficiency symptoms can be reversed by returning linoleic acid to the diet.

Linolenic acid, an omega-3 essential fatty acid, is very important for human health. We cannot make this fatty acid from other fats in our diet. Signs of deficiency of linolenic acid include:

- growth retardation
- weakness
- impairment of vision and learning ability
- motor uncoordination
- tingling sensations in arms and legs
- behavioral changes

These symptoms can be reversed by restoring linolenic acid to the diet. Other symptoms that can result from linolenic acid deficiency include:

- high triglycerides
- high blood pressure
- sticky platelets
- tissue inflammation
- edema (water retention)
- dry skin
- mental deterioration
- low metabolic rate (making it more difficult to lose weight
- immune dysfunction

These symptoms respond very well to addition of linolenic acid to the diet. Deficiencies in linolenic acid are more widespread than formerly believed.[3]

Olive oil also contains saturated fatty acids. Palmitic acid ranges from 7.5 percent to 18 percent (average 10 percent) of the fatty acid content. Palmitic acid is known to raise cholesterol levels, yet olive oil protects arteries rather than damaging them. It may be that the ability of the antioxidant components and oleic acid counteract the effect of palmitic acid. Cholesterol that is protected from oxidation is not a risk factor (see below). The amount of stearic acid which neither raises nor lowers cholesterol levels is, about 2 percent of total fatty acid content.

LDL CHOLESTEROL: NOT SO BAD AFTER ALL

Cholesterol, just like any other fatty compound, can become oxidized. Similarly, it can also be protected from oxidation by the antioxidant vitamins. There is really no such entity as "bad" cholesterol. If cholesterol itself was a harmful substance, it would not be used in our bodies for numerous biochemical and structural tasks such as a starting product for hormone production or a component of the walls of the cells in our bodies.

What is termed "bad" cholesterol is really just unprotected LDL cholesterol. The role of LDL is to carry cholesterol through the blood vessels. Some of this cholesterol migrates into the blood vessel walls, a natural, ongoing process. If there is too much LDL cholesterol or oxidized LDL cholesterol is present, too much of it is taken up into the cells lining the blood vessel walls (called endothelial cells). At high levels, the cholesterol is toxic and causes inflammation of the blood vessel walls. This sets the stage for other biochemical changes that ultimately result in clogged arteries.

There is increasing evidence that oxidatively modified LDL can promote the development of atherosclerosis. Research done at the Rambam Medical Center in Haifa, Israel indicates that an oleic acid-rich diet can reduce the susceptibility of LDL cholesterol to oxidation.[4] A significant reduction in susceptibility to oxidation occurred after only one week of supplementation with olive oil. Macrophage uptake of LDL was reduced after one or two weeks on the olive oil diet. Macrophages are cells in the body's scavenging system. Uptake of LDL by these cells is associated with the formation of atherosclerotic deposits in the blood vessels. The enrichment of the LDL cholesterol with oleic acid and sitosterol from olive oil lowers the ability of LDL to produce atherosclerosis.

Olive oil contains vitamin E, as mentioned earlier. Vitamin E (alpha-tocopherol) has been shown to reduce LDL oxidation in healthy men.[5] Other researchers have found that vitamin E lowers the risk of coronary heart disease.[6]

Other studies have shown that beta-carotene—we noted earlier that it is present in olive oil—can also reduce cardiac events among men with atherosclerotic heart disease. When olive oil is added to the diet it also enriches the LDL molecule with oleic acid and sitosterol, both of which make the LDL more resistant to oxidation. The nutrients in olive oil work in concert to protect LDL cholesterol from oxidation. LDL cholesterol that is thus protected is not "bad" as previously believed by the scientific community.

OLIVE OIL AND DISEASE: RESEARCH CONFIRMS TRADITION

Ancient wisdom on the health benefits of olive oil is being validated by modern research studies. The beneficial effects of olive oil have been demonstrated in the prevention of cardiovascular diseases and breast cancer, in proper functioning of the digestive system, and in treating arthritis.

HEART DISEASE

Olive oil beneficially affects cholesterol levels, blood pressure, blood clotting and protects against atherogenesis.

There is evidence that the Mediterranean diet (see section, "Olive Oil in the Diet") has an important and beneficial effect on the rate of occurrence of coronary heart disease (CHD). In the 1950s a classic international study was done by Ancel Keys, inventor of the U.S. Army K ration (the food that soldiers eat in the field). Keys compared diet and rates of heart disease among seven different countries. He found the least heart disease on the Greek islands of Crete and Corfu, where the largely rural population ate little meat, lots of grains, fruit, and vegetables, and very large quantities of olive oil. The Cretan islanders' daily diet contained as much as 40 percent of calories from olive oil. It was reported that people there drank a glass of olive oil for breakfast.[7]

The study involved over 12,000 middle-aged men and lasted for 30 years. One of the most significant results was that people from Italy and Greece had lower mortality rates than those from northern Europe, America and Japan. Several aspects of the Greek diet that may contribute to its beneficial role in countering the development of CHD were found: high intake of olive oil that lowers LDL cholesterol levels, the regular consumption of fiber-rich legumes and vegetables cooked in olive oil, the high intake of vegetables and fruits with antioxidants, and moderate consumption of wine with meals that raises HDL cholesterol.[8]

During the early period of the Keys study, relatively little attention was paid to HDL cholesterol levels, or to other important components of the Greek or other variants of the Mediterranean diet apart from their low levels of saturated fats. Gradually, despite the original views of Keys's group, Mediterranean diets came to be regarded as healthy simply on account of their low saturated-fat content. The ratio of monounsaturated to saturated fat in the Greek diet is about 2:1.

A look at the consumption of ten selected food items by the population of Athens shows that olive oil was at the top of the list of foods used every day:

Athenians' Top 10 Foods

Food	Percentage of people eating the food at least once every day
olive oil	94.9
bread	94.1
sugar	88.1
uncooked tomatoes	86.6
cheeses	71.6
apples	60.5
cucumbers	57.9
milk	50.8
pears	50.0
onions	37.2
margarine	10.0

The intake of margarine is traditionally low among Greeks, who continue to favor olive oil.

Study findings during the past ten years have provided further evidence of the beneficial effect of the traditional Greek diet on the rate of occurrence of CHD. The beneficial effects of the diet hold even though tobacco consumption and salt intake are high among the Greeks. The health advantages enjoyed by Greek men decrease, however, as they move away from their traditional diet and food culture.

Eating the way your ancestors ate makes a lot of sense. This idea will be further discussed in the section "Food Pyramid or Greek Column?"

Researchers looking for an explanation of the health benefits of olive oil examined the effects of compounds extracted from extra-virgin olive oil.[9] These compounds, called phenols, have antioxidant properties. One in particular, DHPE (2-(3,4-di-hydroxyphenyl)-ethanol) was shown to inhibit platelet function, preventing blood clotting. Several other compounds in the olive oil such as oleuropein (a phenol) and luteolin, apigenin and quercetin (flavonoids) had similar activity against platelets, but to a lesser degree. Oleuropein, the bitter principle of olives, has also been shown to inhibit oxidation of LDL cholesterol, an event implicated in the development of atherogenic disease.[10]

The Jerusalem Nutrition Study looked at the effects of diets rich in monounsaturated fatty acids, including those from olive oil, on cholesterol levels. Healthy normal male college students were put on diets for 12 weeks. The diets consisted of natural and common food items prepared and cooked in customary ways.

In one diet group, following the MUFA diet, fat was added in the form of olive oil, avocado and almonds. In the carbohydrate group, the diet was supplemented with carbohydrate-rich food items. Even when the diets of test subjects contained the same amounts of saturated and polyunsaturated fatty acids, substituting MUFA for carbohydrates was found to have a beneficial effect.[11]

Total plasma cholesterol decreased significantly (about 7.7 percent) and LDL cholesterol decreased by 14.4 percent in persons on the MUFA diet, while on the carbohydrate diet no significant change in cholesterol concentrations occurred. Also, on the MUFA diet, there was a significantly lower proneness to peroxidation of fatty acids and less uptake of LDL cholesterol by macrophages (both processes known to contribute to atherosclerosis).

A study of sedentary middle-aged American men, aged 30 to 55, was conducted to determine the effect on a relatively high intake of monounsaturated fat as olive oil on high blood pressure. The researchers found that higher levels of monounsaturated dietary fat were associated with lower blood pressure, both systolic and diastolic.[12] The monounsaturated fat responsible for this lowering of blood pressure was determined to be oleic acid, the major fatty acid in olive oil. In another study, a blood pressure-lowering effect was also found with diets rich in oleic acid.[13]

Dietary guidelines for the prevention and treatment of coronary heart disease were developed by the Expert panel of the National Cholesterol Education Program.[14] These recommendations clearly state that oleic acid should be the major fatty acid in the diet.

When people who had already had a myocardial infarction (heart attack) were put on diets that contained less saturated fat, cholesterol, and linoleic acid but more oleic and alpha-linolenic acids, they were protected against further heart attacks.[15] Another group of patients who had had heart attacks continued a regular diet. After 27 months, there were 16 deaths from heart attack in the group on the regular diet and three in the group receiving the higher levels of oleic and alpha-linolenic acids. Olive oil, which contains these two fatty acids, was a part of the diet. The outcome was better for the people with diets that included the beneficial fatty acids, even though there were more smokers in this group.

BREAST CANCER

The American Cancer Society's *Cancer Facts and Figures* (1995) states that of the ten most deadly women's cancers, only lung cancer is more deadly than breast cancer. Breast cancer, however is by far the most common cancer in American women. The link between fat in the diet and development of breast cancer is still controversial. In countries with high-fat diets, however, more women have breast cancer. It is known that women in Mediterranean countries, if they are eating traditional diets, have a lower incidence of breast cancer. Olive oil, a major dietary fat in these countries, has been shown to decrease the risk of breast cancer.

Results from a study reported in the *Journal of the National Cancer Institute*, January 18, 1995,[16] indicate that olive oil may even prevent breast cancer. A look at the diets and the rate of breast cancer in 2,368 women (820 with breast cancer and 1548 without) in Greece suggests that women who used olive oil more than once a day had a 25 percent lower risk of breast cancer than women who used that fat less often. Greek women who got 42 percent of their energy intake from fat (mostly olive oil), have substantially lower mortality from breast cancer than U.S. women, whose energy intake from fat is about 35 percent.

Previous studies did not examine the role of margarine consumption in the etiology of breast cancer. In this Greek study, margarine intake appeared to be associated with an elevated risk of breast cancer. Margarine contains trans fatty acids and partially hydrogenated oils, both known to be harmful to the body (see above).

"I wouldn't suggest replacing fats with just any monounsaturated fats," says study coauthor Dimitrios Trichopoulos, M.D., of the Harvard School of Public Health. "There may be something more in olive oil." Dr. Trichopoulos also said that

American women might actually have as much as a 50 percent reduction in breast cancer risk if they consumed more olive oil. He said that even the Greek women who consumed the least olive oil were still taking much more than the highest consumers of the oil in the United States.

As part of a population-based case-control study of the effects of diet on breast cancer, 762 women in Spain, aged 18-75 years, and with breast cancer, were questioned about their diets. Another 988 women without breast cancer were also included. The study found that neither total fat intake nor specific types of fat were significantly associated with breast cancer in pre- or postmenopausal women. However it was found that higher consumption of olive oil (rich in monounsaturated fat) was significantly related to a lower risk of breast cancer. There was a significant dose-response trend in this study (the higher the level of olive oil in the diet, the lower the risk of breast cancer).[17]

Leonard Cohen, a scientist with the American Health Foundation, believes that the diets of Americans are all so fatty that protection against breast cancer would not be noticed with small decreases in total dietary fat. Cohen advised his own wife to "keep fat to 20 percent of calories, to eat more beans, and to cook in olive oil," to reduce her risk of breast cancer. He made this statement because it is known that olive oil does not promote tumors, while corn and other polyunsaturated vegetable oils do.[18]

To reduce the risk of breast cancer, the Center for Science in the Public Interest recommends: "Cut back on the saturated and trans fats that increase your risk of heart disease. When you use oil, stick with olive."

Although it is known that a high-fat diet, no matter what the type of fat, is an important risk factor for the development of breast cancer, fat type may still make a difference. Some studies have indicated that MUFA may be less likely to promote tumors than either saturated or polyunsaturated fatty acids. These studies found that the amount of the essential fatty acid, linoleic acid (LA), correlated with tumor incidence. Oils containing higher levels of LA, which is needed in only small amounts in the diet, were more likely to promote tumors or enlarge tumors in mice.

The researchers found that among mice fed high-fat diets, those who had more LA in their diets (the corn and safflower-oil-fed groups) experienced enhanced development of breast tumors and higher levels of prostaglandin E2 in tumor tissue. This was not the case for the low-LA oils, coconut and olive oil. Just what was the mechanism of tumor promotion? It was found that in groups fed the high-fat olive oil or coconut oil diets, LA was converted faster to prostaglandin precursors than when the diet contained higher levels of LA. But why was there a lower level of prostaglandin in the olive oil-fed group even though conversion is faster?

The results indicated that oleic acid, the chief fatty acid in olive oil, may have exerted its own inhibiting action on prostaglandin synthesis.[19] The researchers concluded that the type of fat was clearly a key determinant of the fat effect. In these animal models, olive oil, because of its low LA content and its apparent inhibitory effect on tumor prostaglandin, was thought to be associated with lower breast cancer risk.

ARTHRITIS

In addition to heart disease, research is now being conducted on the effects of olive oil consumption on rheumatoid arthritis. It was found that patients with the disease consumed significantly less olive oil (and fish oil) than individuals who had less of these nutrients in their diets. In the U.S., a long-term study is now being conducted by the National Arthritis Foundation, to determine the effects of olive oil supplementation on patients with arthritis. The study is being conducted at the University Hospital Arthritis Awareness Center in Coral Springs, Florida. This is the first time in the organization's history that they will be investigating a nontraditional approach for the treatment of arthritis. Additional details of the study are given in the section "Green Gold Goodness to Purified Perfection."

Studies show that omega-3 fatty acids can reduce pain in patients with active rheumatoid arthritis.[20] Olive oil contains omega-3 fatty acids (see above). Olive oil also contains oleic acid which is known to increase the incorporation of omega-3 fatty acids into cell membranes.

In another study it was found that people with rheumatoid arthritis consumed significantly less olive oil and fish than people without the disease. An increase in olive oil consumption by two times per week resulted in a decreased risk of development of rheumatoid arthritis.[21]

DIGESTIVE FUNCTION

Olive oil reduces the severity of ulcers, has a positive effect on the gallbladder and prevents constipation.

Since ancient times, olive oil has been recommended as a

protective agent in cases of gastritis and gastroduodenal ulcers. The use of olive oil, rich in oleic acid, instead of other dietary fats has been shown to reduce ulcer lesions. Fats act on the sphincter muscle that separates the stomach and esophagus. Most edible fats reduce the tonus (muscle tone) of this muscle, causing gastric reflux (heartburn). The muscle is least affected by olive oil and effects last a shorter time than for other oils. Butter is the least tolerated fat, while sunflower oil has intermediate effects. The emptying time of the stomach is affected in the same way by these three fats.

Olive oil also has beneficial effects on the gallbladder. It encourages gallbladder contraction and bile emptying and improves the function of the badly toned, poorly-working gallbladder. Olive oil has a more gentle and prolonged action than prescription drugs and other foods with similar effects. By activating bile flow, olive oil reduces the incidence of gallstones. Olive oil also inhibits hepatic (liver) bile secretion during gallbladder emptying time, thus giving the gallbladder time to empty completely and allowing the bile to work more effectively in emulsifying fats. The ability of olive oil to raise HDL cholesterol also decreases formation of cholesterol-containing gallstones since HDL cholesterol is more easily metabolized to bile acids that are excreted from the body. A long-standing remedy for chronic constipation is two tablespoons of olive oil taken in the morning on an empty stomach.

Some of the minor components in olive oil have been found to have beneficial effects on gastrointestinal function. Caffeic and gallic acids stimulate the flow of bile. Bile secretion improves elimination of the toxic end products of liver detoxification and improves digestion of fats. Another compound found in olive oil, 2-phenylethanol, stimulates production of fat-digesting enzymes in the pancreas. Triterpenic acids (oleanolic and maslinic—found only in olive oil) also stimulate these pancreatic enzymes. Cycloartenol, stored in the liver, lowers the amount of circulating cholesterol and increases bile excretion (in animal studies).

DIABETES

For people who have non-insulin-dependent diabetes mellitus (NIDDM), there is no consensus about the optimal diet. High-carbohydrate, low-fat diets are recommended for these patients and are reported to reduce LDL cholesterol levels. However, other studies suggest that a high-carbohydrate diet may elevate triglycerides, reduce HDL ("good") cholesterol, and may worsen high blood sugar and/or raise plasma insulin levels. These tendencies already exist in NIDDM patients and the recommended diet could aggravate these conditions.

There is some recent evidence that diets high in monounsaturated fats may be of more benefit to NIDDM patients. One recent study was designed to compare the relative long-term effects of substituting monounsaturated fats for carbohydrates on glucose, insulin and lipoprotein levels in people with NIDDM. The study was a four-center, randomized, crossover trial conducted with 42 NIDDM patients, receiving lipizide therapy. One diet contained 55 percent of total energy as carbohydrates and 30 percent as fat. The other diet was high in monounsaturated fats (45 percent) with 40 percent carbohydrates.[22] The amounts of saturated fats, polyunsaturated fats, cholesterol, sucrose and protein were similar in both diets.

Results showed that compared with the high-monounsaturated fat diet, the high-carbohydrate diet increased fasting plasma triglyceride levels, glucose, and insulin values, causing persistent deterioration of diabetic control. The effects of both diets lasted for 14 weeks.

OLIVE OIL IN THE DIET

The answer is "the Mediterranean Diet."

The question is, "What do people in Italy, Greece, Spain, Israel, Egypt, Morocco and other Middle East countries have in common?" One collective practice of these diverse peoples is a diet rich in olive oil—and they reap the health benefits. Butter may be better than margarine, but olive oil is the best dietary fat. A Greek column may be a better food guide model than an Egyptian pyramid.

WHEN IN GREECE

The traditional Greek diet is strongly inversely related to the risk of developing coronary heart disease. Greeks follow what is called the Mediterranean diet. There is good evidence that this diet has important and beneficial effects on the rate of occurrence of CHD as well as on other disease states. Olive oil is the backbone of the Mediterranean diet, providing a larger number of calories than any other single food.

I mentioned earlier the study begun in the 1950s by Dr. Ancel Keys and colleagues in which they followed the health of 12,000 middle-aged men in seven different countries for 30 years. One of the most significant results of the study was that mortality rates were lower for Greek men than for northern European, American and Japanese groups. The difference was especially striking for CHD.

In the early 1980s researchers studied the dietary intake of 14 Mediterranean countries—Portugal, Spain, France, Italy, Yugoslavia, Greece, Malta, Israel, Libya, Algeria, Tunisia, Turkey, Egypt, and Morocco—and found a common nutritional profile (perhaps the only time that these countries were in agreement with each other in any way). Diets in these countries were characterized by a low intake of saturated fat, moderate intake of total fat, mainly monounsaturated (olive oil), and high intake of complex carbohydrates.

The Greek version of the Mediterranean diet was especially considered optimal because life expectancy in Greece was higher than in the U.S. and heart disease and total cancers were less prevalent. The traditional Greek diet is low in saturated fat, high in monounsaturated fat, namely olive oil, high in complex carbohydrates from grains and legumes and high in fiber—mostly from vegetables (cooked in olive oil) and fruits. The high content of fresh fruits and vegetables and cereal and liberal use of olive oil ensure a high intake of beta-carotene, vitamin C, tocopherols, many minerals and other phytonutrients such as polyphenols and proanthocyanadins. Moderate intake of wine was also considered a positive factor.

Greeks also eat more fish and less meat and fewer eggs than U.S. populations. There are few factors other than diet that can explain the remarkable health advantages enjoyed by Greek men (and to a lesser extent, women) in the 1960s and 1970s. The frequency and intensity of smoking of Greek men are among the highest in the world, intentional physical exercise is rarely practiced in Greece (much of the population is rural, however and individuals are not usually sedentary), and there are no nationwide programs for early detection and effective treatment of high blood pressure. The advantage decreases, however, as Greeks change their traditional diet and food culture.

During the past ten years, several research findings have increased the credibility of the reports of the effect of diet on CHD in Greeks. Studies have determined that high levels of HDL cholesterol, moderate drinking of alcoholic beverages, intake of fiber and fruit and vegetables all decrease the risk of CHD. Also, strong evidence that partially hydrogenated vegetable fats (margarine and vegetable shortening) increase CHD, and the fact that Greeks eat very little margarine, provide further evidence of a dietary cause and effect.

Although other factors such as the relaxing psychological environment, the stress-releasing habit of taking afternoon siestas, preservation of the extended family structure, and even mild climatic conditions, may complement the beneficial effects of the traditional diet, the Greek diet is still the central factor in lowering the risk of CHD. Although the average Greek obtains 40 percent of dietary calories from fat, considerably above the "under 30 percent level" recommended in the U.S., this population has had and still has one of the longest life expectancies of all nationalities.

Other studies, evaluating the diet of Greek women, found that higher intakes of vegetables and fruits correlated with significant reduction in breast cancer risk. There was also evidence that olive oil consumption reduced breast cancer while margarine was associated with an elevated risk for the disease. In another study on diet and breast cancer in Spain, higher consumption of olive oil was significantly related to a lower risk of breast cancer.

FOOD PYRAMID OR GREEK COLUMN?

Many countries have developed their own food guides or "pyramids." A common theme for these guidelines is recommendation of lower fat, saturated fat and cholesterol; less salt and sugar; and more fresh fruits and vegetables. In each country, the composition of the pyramid is based on that country's traditional diet: the Mexican (or Mayan) pyramid is based on fruits, vegetables and whole grains. Oriental-type guidelines are based on rice and vegetables.

According to Dr. Artemis P. Simopoulos, President of the Center for Genetics, Nutrition and Health, the ideal food guide is based on the dietary patterns that people had early in the

The USDA Food Guide Pyramid

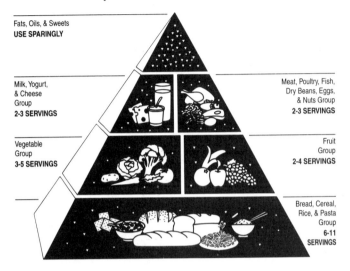

Source: U.S. Department of Agriculture/U.S. Department of Health and Human Services.

evolutionary history of that population. Eating the way your ancestors ate makes sense. It took thousands of years of evolutionary experience to develop the eating patterns of a particular group of people. Although living conditions have changed dramatically over the last 10,000 years, there have been few, if any, changes in our genetic makeup. Our bodies are waiting for the same exercise levels and dietary components that our ancestors adapted to.

According to Dr. Simopoulos, evidence indicates that early diets, dating back to the Paleolithic era, were low in saturated fat and sodium, and higher in protein, antioxidant vitamins, and calcium than current diets. The fat content of these early diets was lower than that of today's Western diet; it was lower in saturated fats and omega-6 fatty acids and higher in omega-3 fatty acids. It also contained minimal amounts of trans fatty acids because these fats rarely occur in nature. Dr. Simopoulos's model for an ideal diet, based on the diet of our early ancestors, is called the Greek column.[23]

The Greek column is based on the food that people of the Mediterranean region ate before 1960, with perhaps more fish

The Greek Column Food Guide

Principles:
- Moderation
- Variety
- Proportionality
- Energy intake = Energy expenditure

} Genetics

Basic components of daily meals

	S	M	T	W	T	F	S
	pasta	fish	legumes	fish	eggs	fish	poultry
	meat	legumes	poultry	legumes	legumes	legumes	legumes

Foods to be added to any meal

olive oil, lemon, vinegar
olives
bread
cheese
yogurt
fruits – fruit juices
nuts, garlic, onions
vegetables, herbs, spices
pasta, rice
water, wine

Source: See Reference 23.

and poultry. Olive oil is the main cooking oil while other vegetable oils and hydrogenated oils are excluded. At the base of the column are foods that can be added to any meal: olive oil, lemon, vinegar, olives. These foods are rich in antioxidant vitamins and minerals and have a balance of omega-6 and omega-3 fatty acids.

There is no limit on how much oil to eat as long as body weight levels are normal. Completing the base are: bread, cheese, yogurt, fruits and fruit juices, nuts, garlic, onions, vegetables, herbs, spices, pasta, rice, potatoes; and water and wine. Above these basic foods, to be consumed in lesser amounts are legumes, fish, and poultry. Meat and eggs are part of a main meal once a week each. There is no place for margarines and other artificial foods. Sweets are eaten rarely or on special occasions, as is true for soft drinks and hard liquor.

The current USDA food guide pyramid has grains as the base, or major dietary platform. It is a high-carbohydrate, low-fat diet, with not enough emphasis on fruits and vegetables. Grains are newcomers to our diet from an evolutionary viewpoint; they only became a staple in our diets about 10,000 years ago. A low-fat diet has been shown in the famous Framingham Study to result in essential fatty acid deficiency in 5 percent to 25 percent of the study population.

Diets high in carbohydrates elevate triglycerides, another contributing factor to heart disease. Our ancestors ate diets high in fruits and vegetables that contained a high content of antioxidant vitamins (vitamins E, C, beta-carotene) and more calcium, folate and fiber. Antioxidants are known to decrease the risk of heart disease, cancer, and prevent or treat many other major diseases.

The most important criticism of the U.S. food pyramid is that it does not distinguish among the various fatty acids, such as trans fatty acids and omega-3 and omega-6 polyunsaturated fatty acids. It does not emphasize the beneficial effects of olive oil in raising HDL cholesterol or in protecting LDL cholesterol from oxidation. The Greek diet is high in monounsaturates. The U.S. diet is high in polyunsaturated fatty acids from vegetable oils rich in omega-6 fatty acids. Such a diet is low in omega-3 fatty acids, creating imbalances that lead to increased tendencies to inflammatory and thrombotic conditions. As use of omega-6 fatty acids increases, prostaglandins and leukotrienes that promote constriction of blood vessels and clotting are made.

Based on the information given, it seems sensible to modify the U.S. food pyramid recommendations. Closer attention to increasing monounsaturated fats and eating as your ancestors ate may make a positive difference in your health.

HOW GOOD IS THE OIL?

This section includes a description of the classifications of olive oil, from "extra virgin" to olive pomace oil and olive oil standards as delineated by the International Olive Oil Council.

How safe and pure is the olive oil sold in the U.S.? According to Richard J. Sullivan, President of the North American Olive Oil Association in Matawan, New Jersey, efforts are being made to assure the purity of olive oil. The Association was set up in cooperation with the International Olive Oil Council, an intergovernmental body under the United Nations supported by government and private trade organizations in the olive oil-producing countries. The North American Olive Oil Association conducts a self-policing program to assure the consumer of the purity of olive oil sold in North America.

The association collects samples of all brands of olive oil from supermarket shelves for testing with advanced analytical methods by laboratories that are specially accredited for the testing of olive oil. These procedures are in accordance with the "Agreement to Monitor the Olive Oils and Olive-Pomace Oils Marketed in the United States and Canada." The Association will provide a copy of this agreement to anyone who requests it. According to the Association, "when a label declares that a product is olive oil, it is a promise that no other food oil is present. To make sure the promise is being kept, we will continue to monitor olive oils sold in the North American market and root out any company that breaks faith with the consumer."

Since olive oil is considered a commodity, it has its own intergovernmental agreement drawn up under the auspices of the United Nations and the United Nations Conference on

Trade and Development (UNCTAD). It is designed to ensure legal guarantees and fair competition in international trade and is administered by the International Olive Council (IOOC) which was created in 1959. Countries that belong to IOOC include Algeria, Cyprus, Egypt, the European Community with its 12 member States, Israel, Morocco, Tunisia, Turkey and the Federal Republic of Yugoslavia.

Most of a sample of olive oil is made up of what is called the saponifiable fraction. This consists of triglycerides and free fatty acids. The major free fatty acid is the monounsaturated oleic acid. The proportions of fatty acid types differ depending on region, olive variety, year and climate, but in general contain the following distribution:

Saturated fatty acids:	8-27 percent
Monounsaturated fatty acids:	55-83 percent
Polyunsaturated fatty acids:	3.5-22 percent

The other fraction of olive oil is known as the unsaponifiable fraction. It is a very small part, but has great biological significance. This fraction contains the chlorophyll which gives a green color, and the carotene content, a reddish pigment, both of which give color to the oil. Also present in this fraction are the polyphenols that account in part for flavor, but are also antioxidants that keep the oils fresh. Tocopherols are also present, mainly vitamin E (alpha-tocopherol, about 10 mg per 100 milliliters of oil), another antioxidant. Sitosterol is the major sterol found. Olive oil contains no cholesterol.

Olive oil mill waste waters were found to be very toxic to several types of bacteria. The compound that proved to have this effect was methylcatechol, a naturally occurring polyphenol in the olive oil.[24] The different grades of olive oil differ in the amount of trans fatty acid content. Edible virgin olive oil contains the least amount (0.03 percent), lampante virgin olive oil contains 0.10 percent. Refined olive oil, olive oil and crude olive-pomace oil all contain 0.20 percent while refined olive-pomace oil and olive-pomace oil contain 0.40 percent. The amount of the trans fatty acids increases with increasing olive oil processing.

The flavor of the oil is partly due to the ripeness of the olive. Green olives picked in September or October have a sharper, fruitier flavor and greener color than the darker, riper olives picked in November and December, which are sweeter and more subtle.

TYPES OF OLIVE OIL

When olives are processed to make oil, several types are obtained. The solid part of the olive paste or mash is called pomace. It contains the bulk of the skin, pulp and pieces of stone and a certain amount of oil.

The general term, "olive oil" means oil obtained solely from the fruit of the olive tree by mechanical means (pressing) and not by the use of solvents or other chemical means. It also excludes mixtures with other types of oils. Olive-pomace oils may not use this term.

The different grades of olive oils and olive-pomace oils are identified by the purity and quality criteria laid down in the IOOC trade standard and are compulsory in international trade.

The very best oils are from olives which are cold-pressed between millstones after drying for two to three days to reduce water content. Small traditional olive oil producers run their mills continuously during the picking season so the olives can be pressed at peak condition. If olives are allowed to sit around, they begin to oxidize (rot), which adversely affects flavor. Larger, commercial production is done with steel plates or by chemical extraction. The heat from some of these larger presses destroys much of the oil flavor, as does the chemical extraction.

The term "virgin" refers to oil obtained from the olive solely by mechanical or other physical means under conditions, particularly thermal conditions, that do not lead to deterioration of the oil. To be designated virgin, the only processes allowed are washing, crushing, preparation of the paste, separation of the solid and liquid phases, decantation and/or centrifugation, and filtration. Virgin olive oil is thus the oily juice of a fruit (the olive). It is virtually the only oil that can be consumed as it comes from the fruit. When properly processed it maintains the flavor, aroma and nutritional components of the fruit.

The legal qualifier for the different grades is the level of acidity. The "first cold-pressed" oils naturally have the least amount of acidity. Oils from the second, third and fourth pressings have much higher acidity and much less flavor. It should be noted that a highly refined, pure olive oil can be "deacidified" and still sold as "extra virgin" (at a much lower cost than real extra virgin). Although this follows the letter of the law, it violates the spirit of it. Regulations may be changed but in the mean time, it would be a good idea to buy olive oil from a grocer you can trust. If a deal on extra virgin oil looks too good to be true, it probably is. Read the labels carefully!

Depending on the criteria it fulfills, olive oils may be called one of the following:

Extra Virgin Olive Oil: a virgin olive oil that has an organoleptic* rating of 6.5 or more and a free acidity, expressed as oleic acid, of not more than 1 gram per 100 grams. This oil is of absolutely perfect flavor, color and aroma and has a maximum acidity of no more than 1 percent. Traditionally, extra virgin was the first pressing of the olives, oil which has been tampered with the least.

Fine Virgin Olive Oil: a virgin olive oil that has an organoleptic rating of 5.5 or more and a free acidity, expressed as oleic acid, of not more than 1.5 grams per 100 grams.

Semi-fine or Ordinary Virgin Olive Oil: a virgin olive oil that has an organoleptic rating of 3.5 or more and a free acidity, expressed as oleic acid, of not more than 3.3 grams per 100 grams.

Lampante Virgin Olive Oil: Virgin olive oil that is not fit for consumption unless it undergoes further processing is known as Lampante Virgin Olive Oil. Lampante means "lamp oil" and it is inedible. It is intended for refining or for technical purposes.

Refined Olive Oil: Obtained from virgin olive oils but not considered suitable for consumption because of high acidity or poor flavor. It must be refined and as a result is without specific color, odor or taste.

Olive Oil: A blend of refined olive oil and virgin olive oil added to achieve a specific taste and to make it fit for consumption. Prior to 1991, this oil was marketed as "Pure Olive Oil," but this name was discontinued based on regulatory changes. The acidity of olive oil is less than 1.5 grams per 100 grams of oil. The taste of these oils differs from one manufacturer to the next.

*Organoleptic is a term that refers to the assessment of virgin olive oil based on the intensity with which the sensorial attributes of a virgin oil are perceived by a panel of 8 to 12 selected, trained tasters who are led by a panel supervisor. Conditions must be met for the type of test room, glasses, temperature of the oil, and specific rules must be followed by the tasters and supervisor. Scores run from zero (clearly perceived, extremely intense defects) to 9, which indicates no defects at all.

Olive Pomace Oil: The oil obtained by treating olive pomace with solvents. It can be:

Crude Olive-Pomace Oil: Intended for refining with a view to its use in food for human consumption, or intended for technical purposes, this oil has no specific taste, color or odor.

Refined Olive-Pomace Oil: Intended for consumption either as it is or in blends with virgin olive oil.

Olive-Pomace Oil: A blend of refined olive-pomace oil and virgin olive oil fit for consumption as it is. In no case whatsoever may it be called "olive oil."

The best way to store olive oil is in an airtight container, away from light in a cool cupboard. Kept this way, it can stay fresh for at least a year. Refrigeration, while not harmful, is not necessary and may make olive oil cloudy and thick. If this happens, just let it warm to room temperature and it will be clear again. Olive oil is best when used within a year of purchase.

It is the flavor of the oil that is rated. Connoisseurs rate olive oil flavors as mild (delicate, light or "buttery"); semi-fruity (stronger, with more taste of the olive); and fruity (oil with full-blown olive flavor). The positive flavor attributes in virgin olive oil are:

- the fruity flavor compared to the odor and taste of sound, fresh olives harvested at their optimum stage of ripeness
- the "bitter," "pungent," "green leaves" and "sweet" attributes which depend on the variety and ripeness of the olives and climatic conditions.

The color of the olive oil does not necessarily indicate how the oil will taste. Color can be affected by growing conditions. Bad-tasting olive oil may result from fermentation of the olives (termed "fusty"), through oxidation ("rancid"), and from the oil coming into contact with vegetable water or tank sediment, or by poor processing.

The terms "first pressing" and "cold pressing" both mean that the olives have been pressed at room temperature to obtain the initial oil/water combination.

Food additives are not permitted for the virgin olive oils and crude olive-pomace oils. For refined olive oil, olive oil, refined olive-pomace oil and olive-pomace oil, addition of alpha-tocopherol (vitamin E) is permitted to restore the natural tocopherol lost in the refining process. The maximum level of alpha-tocopherol allowed in the final product is 200 mg/kg of oil.

Can you always tell where a particular olive oil was produced? Not always. The name of the country of origin should be given. If the oil undergoes processing or repacking, including in small containers, in a second country, it is this country that will be listed. Virgin olive oils that are produced in a region or locality and have been authorized by their country of origin to indicate that source, are usually truthfully labeled. For example, when a bottle label reads "Lucca," that is where the olive oil has been produced, packed and originates from exclusively. The labels for blends of refined olive oil and virgin olive oil may indicate only the exporting country.

The best way to become familiar with the wide range of olive oil flavors is to taste as many types as possible. To save money, consider sharing bottles of the different oils with friends or relatives.

OLIVE OIL AND BAKING

Olive oil has a small fat crystal which yields even, fine textured baked goods. The tocopherols (vitamin E) that act as emulsifiers produce a smooth, homogeneous batter and cakes that have a moist and tender crumb. The tocopherols also act as antioxidants and keep the baked goods fresher longer.

Using olive oil in baking dramatically cuts the cholesterol and saturated fat content. Using olive oil instead of butter produces lighter-tasting baked goods and also allows the flavor of the other ingredients to come through with more clarity.

Examples of baked goods with olive oil are:

- carrot, chocolate, spice and fruit cakes
- cookie bars and brownies
- graham cracker, nut or cookie crusts
- corn bread or sticks and other hot batter breads, muffins and biscuits
  - pancakes, blinis and crepes
  - flat breads, pizza crust

Baking conversions:

Butter/Margarine	Olive oil
1 teaspoon	3/4 teaspoon
1 tablespoon	2 1/4 teaspoons
2 tablespoons	1 1/2 tablespoons
1/4 cup	3 tablespoons
1/3 cup	1/4 cup
1/2 cup	1/4 cup + 2 tbs.
2/3 cup	1/2 cup
3/4 cup	1/2 cup + 1 tbs.
1 cup	3/4 cup

THE EATING OF THE OLIVE

In addition to standards for olive oil production and marketing, there are also a set of rules governing table olives, the fruit itself. When deciding what varieties to use for table processing, each producer country receives recommendations:

- The fruit should be a good size and shape
- It should have a good flesh:stone ratio
- The flesh should be delicate, flavorsome and firm, and the skin should be fine
- The flesh should separate easily from the stone, which should be small and smooth

Once they are selected and packed, table olives must be presented:

- sound and clean
- free from abnormal flavors and odors
- at the right state of ripeness
- devoid of defects liable to affect the edibility or keeping properties
- devoid of any foreign matter except authorized ingredients
- with no sign of any deterioration or any abnormal fermentation
- size-graded and of one variety to a container
- of uniform color, except for seasoned olives and olives turning color

Authorized ingredients that may be optional are: water, salt, vinegar, olive oil, sugars; any product used as stuffing material and prepared pastes of such materials; spices, aromatic herbs and their natural extracts. Ferrous lactate (a form of iron) may be added to darken the fruit. Benzoic, sorbic, lactic, citric and ascorbic (vitamin C) acids are added to preserve the fruit. Sodium hydroxide may be added to decrease acidity.

Brines are edible sodium chloride (salt) solutions in drinkable water, with or without sugar, vinegar or lactic acid, oil and other authorized substances; aromatic spices or plants may be added. When packed in glass bottles, the brines should be clear (transparent).

There are three trade categories for classifying olives:

Extra or Fancy: These are high-quality olives that have the maximum specific characteristics considered to belong to the variety. They may have slight color, shape, firmness or skin defects if these do not affect the overall organoleptic characteristics of the fruit.

First, Choice or Select: This category includes good-quality olives at a suitable degree of ripeness, having the variety's specific characteristics. They may have slight shape, color or firmness defects.

Second or Standard: These olives comply with the general conditions defined although they cannot be classified in the two previous categories.

GREEN GOLD GOODNESS TO PURIFIED PERFECTION

What do you do if you want the health benefits of olive oil but do not like the taste? What if you want therapeutic benefits and need the purest form of olive oil available? Like other fats and oils, olive oil is subject to chemical breakdown. It can become rancid, producing substances such as peroxides and free radicals that may contribute to inflammation, suppression of the immune system and other adverse health conditions. There is an ultra-purification process that produces therapeutic-grade (also called pharmaceutical grade) olive oil. Purification does not alter the fundamental, healthful lipid profile. In the process, impurities present in the oil, such as peroxides and oxidation products are removed by a procedure called column chromatography. Basically, the unwanted impurities in the oil stick to a column of absorbent materials while the purified oil runs through and out of the column. The result is a water-clear, odorless liquid with a low peroxide value. Peroxides can generate free radicals, causing inflammation and tissue damage which can aggravate arthritis and other medical conditions.

Peroxides cause harm to the body in the following ways:

1. They are carcinogenic
2. They suppress the immune system
3. They contribute to inflammation
4. They cause atherosclerosis
5. They are mutagenic (for pregnant women)

The ultra-purified olive oil can be taken in capsules. Because of the refining process, this dosage form is standardized—each capsule contains the same amount of fatty acids and antioxidants. The potency of the oil is consistent and the stability is improved. These properties are important when a nutritional substance is used for therapeutic purposes. If a scientific clinical trial is developed to test the effect of a supplement on a disease condition, the physicians must know exactly how much and what the components are in that supplement. It is also important, both for the researcher and the patients, to know what is not in the supplement—peroxides or other unwanted substances.

The National Arthritis Foundation has been studying the effects of ultra-purified olive oil at the University Hospital Arthritis Awareness Center in Coral Springs, Florida. The study participants include people with rheumatoid arthritis, fibrositis, fibromyalgia or osteoporosis. If the results are encouraging, it will serve as a pilot study and be proposed to the 76 regional branch offices of the Foundation.

OLIVE OIL FACTS

Did you know that:

• People living in the Mediterranean area who use olive oil as their main fat source have the lowest mortality rate due to cardiovascular illness. In the United States and Finland, where people eat high amounts of saturated fat, this mortality rate is the highest.
• Using olive oil in place of saturated fats as the main fat in your diet may actually reduce cholesterol levels.
• Olive oil protects itself from becoming rancid. Rancidity means that the fatty acids in an oil have reacted with oxygen to form peroxides. This process causes the oil to deteriorate in taste and in quality.
• Many cooking oils, those made from seeds and animal fats, become oxidized when used to fry foods. This process produces toxic compounds that can adversely affect body organs. Olive oil, because of its higher natural antioxidant content, does not oxidize as much as the other cooking oils and can be used to fry foods at high temperatures. Olive oil coats food instead of being absorbed. You can fry, stir fry and even deep fry with olive oil. It can be filtered after frying and reused four to five times before being discarded. Other fats and oils can be used only twice.
• If a recipe calls for "olive oil," it is probably best to use regular olive oil or even olive pomace oil for heavy-duty, high-heat cooking. If you want to taste the flavor of the oil, it is best to use virgin olive oils and add the oil to cooked dishes in the final stages.
• Olive oil has the same amount of calories as other cooking oils: 120 calories to a tablespoon (or 9 calories per gram) of oil. Because olive oil has more flavor and aroma than other oils, you will probably use less in cooking or as salad oil. This will help you cut calories!
• "Light" olive oils are not low in fat. They are simply plain

olive oils that have had little or no extra virgin oil added after refining.
- There are over 75 varieties of olives and of the oils produced, no two flavors are alike. No other cooking oil offers such a variety.
- Go to Naples—Dietary antioxidant intake and levels of lipid peroxidation were determined in healthy young persons in Naples (southern Italy) and compared to people in Bristol (U.K.). These people ate typical regional foods. Those from Naples ate more tomatoes and monounsaturated fatty acids from olive oil than their English counterparts. The Italians had lower levels of lipid peroxidation (associated with atherogenesis) in their bodies. Levels of lipid peroxidation are determined by measuring by-products of peroxidation such as dienes and peroxides. The lower levels of peroxidation may contribute to the lower risk of coronary artery disease found in southern Italy.[25]
- Olive oil and sunflower oil are both high in monounsaturated fatty acid. However, when studies were done using both oils, olive oil increased HDL ("good") cholesterol levels by 7 percent while sunflower oil increased it by 4 percent.[26]
- The Bible makes 140 references to olive oil and close to 100 of the olive tree. The Bible is a rich source of information on the religious and culinary uses of olive oil. The Koran speaks of olive oil and Greek and Roman literature is full of references to the olive tree and its produce.
- Throughout the world there are approximately 24,000,000 acres with over 800 million olive trees; 98 percent are located in the Mediterranean countries. Average yearly production is approximately 9,000,000 metric tons, of which 800,000 are table olives.
- The olive products sector generates yearly, approximately 200,000,000 working days, the majority of which are jobs for people of limited incomes.

SUMMARY

As we are being told to reduce our fat intake to less than 30 percent of calories in order to avoid the ravages of heart disease and various kinds of cancer, the research discussed above is demonstrating that it is possible to eat just as much fat as ever, yet remain protected from the chronic diseases that plague so many of us during the last 10 to 20 years of our lives. The key to consumption of fats and oils, as demonstrated in this book, is knowing what type to eat.

Many of us would be more pleased to follow diets that include more fat than the US Dietary Guidelines diet, with its "lean" instructions for choosing a diet low in fat. The composition of fatty acids in olive oil places it at the top of the list when it comes to taste and good health.

RESOURCES

Here are some addresses and phone numbers for further information on olive oil and olive oil products:

The International Olive Oil Council
Contact: Foodcom, Inc.
733 Third Avenue
New York, NY 10017
(212) 297-0136
Fax (212) 297-0139

   The International Olive Oil Council provides a consumer "olive oil hotline," 1-800-232-OLIVE-OIL. Use the letter "O" when dialing "OLIVE" or call 1-800-232-6548. The hotline is open Monday through Friday, 9:00 a.m. to 5:00 p.m., Eastern time. The hotline is staffed by registered dietitians who will answer questions on health-related topics, and provides information on 10,000 branded items found in stores and supermarkets. Free booklets and brochures with recipes and information concerning olive oil can also be obtained.

The hotline services are provided in cooperation with The New York Hospital-Cornell University Medical College Nutrition Information Center under the direction of Barbara Levine, R.D., Ph.D.

Health Products International, Inc.
450 Commack Road
Deer Park, NY 11729
(516) 254-1094
Fax (516) 254-1234
Manufacturer of ultra-purified pharmaceutical grade olive oil.

Nutrition Headquarters
One Nutrition Plaza
Carbondale, IL 62901
1-800-851-3551
Supplier (to consumers) of ultra-purified pharmaceutical grade olive oil.

REFERENCES

1. *Harvard Heart Letter.* Trans-fatty acids: The new enemy, July 1994, Vol. 4, Issue 11, pp. 1-3.
2. Kiritsakis A, Markakis P. Olive oil: a review. *Advances in Food Research.* 1987;31:467-468.
3. Erasmus, U. *Fats that Heal, Fats that Kill.* Burnaby B.C. Canada: Alive Books, 1993.
4. Aviram M, Eias K. Dietary olive oil reduces low-density lipoprotein uptake by macrophages and decreases the susceptibility of the lipoprotein to undergo lipid peroxidation. *Annals of Nutr & Metab.* 1993;37(2):75-4.
5. Jialal I, Fuller CJ, Huet BA. *Arterioscler Thromb Vasc Biol.* 1995;15:190-198.

6. Bays H, Dujovne C. Antioxidants in clinical practice. *Choices in Cardiology.* 1994;8(1):6-8.
7. Keys A. *Seven Countries: A Multivariate Analysis of Death and Coronary Heart Disease.* Cambridge:Harvard University Press; 1980.
8. Trichopoulou A, Lagiou P, Trichopoulos D. Traditional Greek diet and coronary heart disease. *J Cardiovasc Risk.* 1994;1:9-15.
9. Petroni A, Blasevich M, Salami M, Papini N, Montedoro GF, Galli C. Inhibition of platelet aggregation and eicosanoid production by phenolic components of olive oil. *Thromb Res.* 1995;78(2):151-160.
10. Visioli F, Galli C. Oleuropein protects low density lipoprotein from oxidation. *Life Sci.* 1994; 55(24):1965-1971.
11. Berry EM, Eisenberg S, Friedlander Y, et al. Effects of diets rich in monounsaturated fatty acids on plasma lipoproteins—the Jerusalem Nutrition Study. II, Monounsaturated fatty acids vs. carbohydrates. *Am J Clin Nutr.* 1992;56:394-403.
12. Williams PT, Fortmann SP, Terry RB, et al. Associations of dietary fat, regional adiposity, and blood pressure in men. *JAMA.* 1987;257(23)3251-3256.
13. Trevisan M, Kragh V., Freudenheim J. et al. Consumption of olive oil, butter and vegetable oils and coronary heart disease risk factors. *JAMA.* 1990;263:633-692.
14. Report of the National Cholesterol Education Program Expert Panel on Detection, Evaluation and Treatment of High blood cholesterol in adults. *Arch Intern Med.* 1988;148:36-69.
15. de Lorgeril M, Renaud S, Mamelle N et al. Mediterranean alpha-linolenic acid-rich diet in secondary prevention of coronary heart disease. *Lancet.* 1994;343:1454-1459.
16. Trichopoulou A, et al. Consumption of olive oil and specific food groups in relation to breast cancer risk in Greece. *J Natl Cancer Inst.* 1995;87(2):110-116.
17. Martin-Moreno JM, Willett WC, Gorgojo L, et al. Dietary fat, olive oil intake and breast cancer risk. *Int J Cancer.* 1994;58(6):774-780.
18. Breast Cancer. Cover story, *Nutrition Action Healthletter.* Center for Science in the Public Interest. January/February 1996, pp. 4-7.
19. Cohen LA, Thompson DO, Choi K, et al. Dietary fat and mammary cancer. II. Modulation of serum and tumor lipid composition and tumor prostaglandin by different dietary fats: Association with tumor incidence patterns. *JNCI.* 1986;77:43-51.
20. Geusens P, Wouters C, Nijs J, Jiang Y, Dequeker J. Long-term effect of omega-3 fatty acid supplementation in active rheumatoid arthritis. A 12-month, double-blind, controlled study. *Arthritis Rheum.* 1994;37(6):824-829.
21. Linos A, Kaklamanis E, Kontomerkos A, et al. The effect of olive oil and fish consumption on rheumatoid arthritis—a case control study. *Scand J Rheumatol.* 1991;20(6):419-426.
22. Garg A, Bantle J, Henry RR, Coulson A, Griver KA. Effects of varying carbohydrate content of diet in patients with non-insulin dependent diabetes mellitus. *JAMA.* 1994;271:1421-1428.
23. Simopoulos AP. The Mediterranean food guide. Greek column rather than an Egyptian pyramid. *Nutrition Today.* 1995;30(2):54-61.
24. Capasso R, Evidente A, Schivo L, Orru G, Marcialis MA, Cristinzio G. Antibac-

terial polyphenols from olive oil mill waste waters. *J Appl Bacteriol.* 1995;79(4):393-398.
25. Mancini M, Parfitt VJ, Rubba P. Antioxidants in the Mediterranean diet. *Can J Cardiol.* 1995;11(suppl G):105G-109G.
26. Perez J-F, Espino A, Lopez-Segura F et al. Lipoprotein concentrations in normolipidemic males consuming oleic acid-rich diets from two different sources: olive oil and oleic acid-rich sunflower oil. *Am J Clin Nutr.* 1995;62(4):769-775.